The Arthritis Myth

The Arthritis Myth

Your Nonsurgical, Drug-Free Approach to Treating Arthritis

Fadi Al-Selhi, DC

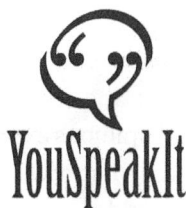

YouSpeakIt

PUBLISHING

The Easy Way
to Get Your Book
Done Right™

www.YouSpeakItPublishing.com

This book is dedicated to my wife Pateala and my son Vincent for their kindness, love, and endless support.

Acknowledgments

First and foremost, I am grateful to God for the blessings he has bestowed upon me to allow me to complete this book.

I thank my wife Pateala, my son Vincent, and the rest of my family for being extremely supportive throughout the long writing journey. I would also like to thank my parents, George and Sawsan Al-Silhi, for their continuous support for everything that I do.

Thank you to all the team members of YouSpeakIt Book Program for enabling me to publish this book.

And, I wish to express my gratitude to all my patients, who give purpose to my life every day.

Contents

Introduction

This book offers a new view on an alternative treatment for the painful, chronic problem of arthritis that is suffered by millions of Americans. It is possible for you to reverse your arthritis without using medications or surgeries or medical procedures.

This book will help you understand:

- What arthritis is
- Different types of arthritis
- Medical standards of care for arthritis
- Your options for treating arthritis outside the U.S. health insurance model

This book will also help you to understand how diet plays a significant role in arthritis. You can take care of your health and promote a better quality of life through proper nutrition. This book will discuss the standards you can use to evaluate your diet and understand why issues such as arthritis, inflammation, and other chronic conditions are increasing in the population year after year.

You will read testimonials by patients who have been in your shoes. These people have been dealing with arthritic pain or inflammation, and they have tried other procedures that did not work for them. Once they implemented the program that I personally designed for them, their arthritis eased, their quality of life improved, and their overall health benefited.

I wrote this book to explain the causes, symptoms, and types of arthritis. There are many people who suffer from joint pain, stiffness, and inflammation, and who unfortunately become discouraged after many different doctors give them the same diagnosis: arthritis. However, these patients are not given a complete understanding of the causes and conditions of arthritis. Understanding what arthritis is and how inflammation plays a role will help you to explore many other options for self-care.

The second reason I wrote this book is to help you understand what alternative treatments are available.

The program that I have designed for arthritis is highly successful. For example, many of my patients did not have to go through surgery. Most doctors will focus on medications, surgeries, and injections for their patients, but there are other ways to address your arthritis, and in my experience these alternatives offer real hope and relief for a great many people.

The final reason I decided to write this book is to help people who suffer from arthritis understand how diet can directly affect their bodies in general, and can increase their arthritis symptoms specifically, because it is an inflammatory condition.

Understanding what our American diet is and comparing it to a good anti-inflammatory diet is very important, because the more you control these factors, the more you will be able to control your condition through:

- Your environment
- What you eat
- Your lifestyle

You will notice how food plays a role and how much better you will feel on an anti-inflammatory diet. With these everyday choices, you have the ability to put your arthritis into remission.

Reading this book, you will gain information that, unfortunately, is usually not discussed or well known to many Americans. Our healthcare model and our standard of care have been focused on only a few treatments for a very long time, and alternative medicine has been frowned upon for many years. There are reasons for this, which we will explore.

In this book, you will learn why alternative medicine is the number-one, go-to medicine at this time, and why many patients are turning toward alternative care practitioners. They are experiencing how alternative medicine helps treat the cause of a problem, as compared to the current standard of care, which focuses on symptoms.

Gathering information and gaining knowledge for your own self-care will empower you. You will never look at healthcare in the same way again. You will not only discard old habits and learn new, helpful ones, but you will also set an example for your friends and family, and be part of a great movement toward alternative medicine.

CHAPTER ONE

What Is Arthritis?

DEFINITION OF ARTHRITIS

Defining arthritis has never been easy for many doctors. All we know about arthritis is that it's caused by inflammation in the joints. However, most doctors believe that arthritis is a normal part of aging. Saying that arthritis occurs naturally with aging is almost the same as saying that inflammation is a normal part of aging. This opens a new argument regarding whether arthritis is inflammatory or not.

The most common type of arthritis is osteoarthritis, or arthritis in the bone. For many years, it was argued that osteoarthritis is noninflammatory. A study that I'm going to be referring to quite a bit in this book is titled, "Is Osteoarthritis a Mechanical or an Inflammatory Disease?"[1]

---

[1] Márcia Uchôa de Rezend and Gustavo Constantino de Campos, "Is Osteoarthritis a Mechanical or an Inflammatory Disease?" © 2013 Sociedad Brasiliera de Ortopedia e Traumaologia. Elsevier Editora Ltd. All rights reserved. Available at: www.scielo.br/scielo.php?script=sci_arttext&pid=S0102-36162013000600471. Accessed Mar. 10, 2017.

The authors state:

> The concept that osteoarthritis (OA) is an inevitable consequence of aging, i.e., wear and tear on the joints due to use, is gradually being left behind. The term "degenerative joint disease," which is still greatly used, denotes the idea of futility and inevitability and does not express the true complexity of the problem.

I will break down the word *arthritis* and give the definition of the word, because once you understand what arthritis really is, you will understand how you can go about treating and managing it. Furthermore, you will understand why other forms of treatment have not worked and why the alternative treatment offered in this book can be a solution for you.

Many Americans are not aware that there are over one hundred types of arthritis. Arthritis does not discriminate against age, race, or sex. The leading cause of disability in the United States is arthritis. In most cases, it can start in a very mild form and then progress. Some studies argue that there is a direct correlation between aging and arthritis; however, lifestyle can be a factor as well.

Now that you have a more complete understanding of what arthritis is, let's take a closer look at how inflammation plays a role in arthritis, and why symptoms tend to worsen with time.

Arthritis Is an Inflammatory Condition

The word *arthritis* is a combined form of two words. The first part of the word is *arth-*, which means *joint*. The second part of the word is *-itis*, which means *inflammation*. *Arthritis* is inflammation in one or more of your joints; therefore, it is an inflammatory condition. Most of the pain that patients feel in their body or joints is from inflammation.

Inflammation is responsible for:

- Pain
- Decreased mobility
- Decreased range of motion
- Swelling

Some studies found that patients who suffer from osteoarthritis have elevated levels of inflammatory *cytokines* in serum and the synovial fluid. Cytokines are small proteins that are responsible for sending signals to the cells. The following excerpt shows the abstract of the study by de Rendez and de Campos, which offers an overview of what will be discussed in the next section.

> Traditionally considered a "wear and tear" disease, the pathogenic mechanisms of osteoarthritis have not yet been elucidated. The increasing number of articles demonstrating the influence of inflammatory factors in the onset and progression of the disease currently raises great debate in the literature about the importance of each of the factors involved in the disease. Even the choice between the terms "Osteoarthritis" and "Osteoarthrosis" generates controversy, since the first term implies the presence of inflammation as the key generator of the disease, and the latter denotes a degenerative/mechanical causal factor. The aim of this revision article is to promote a debate on the influence of inflammatory factors and mechanical factors in the pathogenesis of OA.[2]

When chronic inflammation is present, it impedes circulation and delivery of nutrients to the tissues.

---

[2]Ibid.

Therefore, this leads to a stage of degeneration in the tissues.

Other studies argue that there are clinical symptoms of *synovitis* — or local inflammation of the synovial membrane — associating the condition with osteoarthritis. Synovitis can be detected by magnetic resonance imaging (MRI). This procedure is often done with contrast and ultrasonography (US), as well, and these methods are great tools in the study of synovitis.

Cartilage deterioration progresses when *joint effusion* — a condition in which there is too much fluid in the joint — and synovitis are present. Loss of cartilage therefore promotes degeneration of the joint, or osteoarthritis.

For a long time, doctors have argued whether arthritis is inflammatory. If it is an inflammatory disease, then it isn't a normal part of aging. Many doctors argue that inflammation is not necessarily a normal part of aging. Certainly, we can agree that people tend to lose some cartilage or disc space due to age, but it doesn't have to be painful or inflammatory. Pain is not initiated from loss of cartilage; in fact, stiffness is one of the first common symptoms of arthritis due to loss of cartilage. Pain is a symptom of inflammation.

Another review, titled "Osteoarthritis and Cartilage," examines an inflammatory component of osteoarthritis and concludes that it's not merely a mechanical effect. I would like to share with you the abstract of this review to expand our understanding.

OA used to be considered the sole consequence of any process leading to increased pressure on one particular joint or fragility of cartilage matrix. Progress in molecular biology in the 1990s has profoundly modified this paradigm. The discovery that many soluble mediators such as cytokines or prostaglandins can increase the production of matrix metalloproteinases by chondrocytes led to the first steps of an "inflammatory" theory. However, it took a decade before synovitis was accepted as a critical feature of OA, and some studies are now opening the way to consider the condition a driver of the OA process. Recent experimental data have shown that subchondral bone may have a substantial role in the OA process, as a mechanical damper, as well as a source of inflammatory mediators implicated in the OA pain process and in the degradation of the deep layer of cartilage. Thus, initially considered cartilage driven, OA is a much more complex disease with inflammatory mediators released by cartilage, bone and synovium. Low-grade inflammation induced by the metabolic syndrome, innate immunity and inflaming are some of the more recent arguments in favor of the inflammatory theory of OA and highlighted in this review.[3]

Arthritis Is Degenerative

Remember, osteoarthritis is also known as *degenerative joint disease*. The term degenerative suggests that this process will get worse with time. Arthritis is an inflammatory condition, and most inflammatory conditions tend to worsen, especially as we age. When chronic inflammation exists, most patients notice their symptoms progress, and the loss of motion in the joint is more pronounced over time.

Many of my patients notice that what they are suffering from today, or the symptoms they are experiencing

[3]Francis Berenbaum, "Osteoarthritis and Cartilage" © 2012 Osteoarthritis Research Society International. Published by Elsevier Ltd. All rights reserved.

now, have progressed from the moment when the pain began a few weeks, months, or years ago:

- Balance is not what it used to be
- Weakness in the joints has increased
- Muscles are becoming atrophied
- Pain changes from a dull ache to sharp, shooting pains

For example, when arthritis progresses in the spine, neck, or lower back, the nerves become more pinched and inflamed over time, which introduces new symptoms such as:

- Numbness
- Tingling
- Burning
- Sharp, shooting pains
- Weakness

Most inflammatory conditions are classified as degenerative. However, there is hope: there are treatments we can take, and there are self-care regimens we can follow to slow down the progression of arthritis, stop it from progressing any further, or even put arthritis into remission.

The Epidemiology of Arthritis

In the United States, between the years 2010 and 2012, about 52.5 million adults were told by their doctors that they had some sort of arthritis, whether it was osteoarthritis, rheumatoid arthritis, gout, or fibromyalgia. More and more people are being diagnosed with these conditions. As healthcare practitioners, we need to educate our patients thoroughly about what arthritis is and what the proper forms of treatment may be.

Many patients suffering from arthritis are told that there is not much that can be done, or that they must simply live with it, or that surgery will be needed. This is especially true for people with knee pain who are advised to get knee replacements, even though these replacements are only a temporary solution. One of two people may develop symptomatic knee arthritis.

If you know the symptoms and types of arthritis, it helps you realize there is something you can do, and you can take actions to slow the progress or stop it altogether, so it does not reach a more degenerative state.

THE PHYSIOLOGY OF ARTHRITIS

Arthritis plays a role in affecting your nervous system.

What Happens in Arthritis?

The most common type of arthritis is osteoarthritis. *Osteo-* comes from the Greek word *osteon*, meaning *bone*, and *osteoarthritis* is the combined word meaning *arthritis in the bone*.

Osteoarthritis is a degeneration or breakdown of articular cartilage, which is cartilage that forms in between the joints. The loss of the cartilage makes the joint *hypomobile*, meaning a lack of motion, or a decrease in range of motion of the joint, due to the fact that the bones are closer together. Therefore, the first and most common symptom that arthritis patients experience is morning stiffness, which gradually improves throughout the day.

The deterioration or breakdown of the articular cartilage, causing the bones to come closer together, initiates a process of inflammation and irritation. With inflammation, most patients experience further clinical symptoms, such as swelling, pain, and decreased mobility.

How Circulation Plays a Role in Arthritis

Because arthritis ends with *-itis*, which means *inflammation*, there is a general rule that explains the condition. Wherever there is an area of inflammation, there is a lack of circulation. If there is some arthritis in the neck or in the lower back, and there is inflammation, it means there is not enough blood flow in that area.

One of the problems with inflammation is that every single tissue in your body is a living tissue:

- Cartilage
- Bones
- Nerves
- Muscles

All living tissues need blood circulation because this is how these cells get their oxygen, nutrients, food, and water. When there is a lack of circulation, that area will continue to degenerate. The treatment that we focus on basically addresses how to bring circulation back to the area so that you can stop the progression of degeneration and get rid of the inflammation that is taking over.

The Effects on the Nervous System

When arthritis occurs in the spine, it may be diagnosed as:

- Osteoarthritis
- Degenerative joint disease
- Degenerative disc disease

Most people have seven vertebrae in the neck, which is known as the *cervical spine*. There are twelve in the upper and mid-back, known as the *thoracic spine,* and five vertebrae in the lower back, known as the *lumbar spine*.

The spinal column houses the spinal cord, which extends from the brain down to the top lumbar vertebra, L1, or the second one, L2. At almost every level in the spine there are nerves that branch out. The nerves that branch out from the cervical spine travel down through your shoulders, arms, and forearms, into your fingers. The nerves that branch out from the lower back, or the lumbar spine, go down the buttocks, thigh, legs, and into the feet and toes.

When a process of degeneration or arthritis takes place in the spine, the spaces that the nerves branch out from start to close, which puts pressure on the nerves.

Common symptoms of nerve compression include:

- Numbness, tingling, or burning sensations
- Sharp, shooting pain or stabbing pain
- Coordination problems
- Balance problems

Some patients report these symptoms as *sciatica*, characterized by pain, tingling, or numbness that can extend down the leg to the big toe. Others can be diagnosed with *radiculopathy*, or *neuropathy* — or conditions caused by compressed nerves — which can be complications of arthritis. Often, we see these conditions as having a direct effect on the nervous system and on the messages that travel from certain body parts to the brain.

One of the biggest problems that can be encountered with severe osteoarthritis in the lumbar spine is balance. An early symptom of balance problems that most patients notice is having a hard time taking a step when standing after prolonged sitting. Most patients report feeling off-balance, or needing to wait a minute or two before taking the next step forward.

Because these nerves do not work optimally, the brain takes longer to recognize where the feet are.

This phenomenon is known as *kinesthetic awareness*, or proprioception, in which your brain can tell where your body is in space at all times. However, when the nerves don't work as well, the brain has a harder time or takes longer to read where the body is, which causes a delay in taking the next step.

Balance issues can progress to falls, or to the need for an assisted walking device, such as a cane, walker, or wheelchair.

Muscle weakness is another problem. In order to work properly, muscles receive an electrical stimulus from nerves. Symptoms occur when the nerves do not fire the proper stimuli that are needed for the muscles to contract properly. This often causes weakness in the extremities and can also contribute to loss of balance if nerves in the lower extremity are affected.

Arthritis patients experiencing these muscle troubles may complain or show signs of:

- Cramps
- Spasms
- Atrophy
- Weakness

THE DIFFERENT TYPES OF ARTHRITIS

It's important to understand the different types of arthritis, because you want to know what type of arthritis you have and how it should be treated. We only hear of osteoarthritis and rheumatoid arthritis because those two are the most common. However, there are over one hundred types of arthritis altogether. Once you understand the type of arthritis you are dealing with, you will understand the symptoms that you are feeling and how you should go about getting it treated.

There's been an argument for years that the main types of arthritis are inflammatory and noninflammatory. However, recent studies have shown that even osteoarthritis should be classified as an inflammatory arthritis because inflammation plays such a large role in osteoarthritis.

Osteoarthritis

Osteoarthritis is also known as *degenerative joint disease.* You will also hear it referred to as *wear-and-tear arthritis.* The *Merck Manual of Diagnosis and Therapy* defines osteoarthritis as "a chronic arthropathy of an entire joint characterized by disruption and potential loss of joint cartilage along with other joint changes, including bone hypertrophy (osteophyte formation)" (*Merck Manual*, 19th ed.).

Osteoarthritis is the most common type of arthritis and is a chronic condition that affects the joints. The cartilage between the joints, which we also call the *cushion*, starts to break down. The loss of cartilage brings the bones closer together, which causes stiffness and can possibly lead to inflammation, which will generate pain and swelling.

We know that there are several possible factors that cause osteoarthritis:

- Previous work injuries
- Previous car accidents
- Lifestyle
- Physically demanding jobs

The most common forms of treatment are:

- Weight management
- Physical therapy
- Pain medications

When it progresses to a certain extent, it can possibly lead to surgery.

The Difference Between Osteoarthritis and Rheumatoid Arthritis

One of the biggest differences between osteoarthritis and rheumatoid arthritis is that rheumatoid arthritis is a chronic inflammatory disorder that affects mainly the hands. It can occur in the knees and the hips, but is most common in the hands.

Rheumatoid arthritis is an autoimmune disease, and therefore can affect other parts of the body:

- Skin
- Lungs
- Eyes
- Heart
- Blood vessels

Rheumatoid arthritis affects 1 percent of the population, and is most common in middle-aged women.

Osteoarthritis is seen more often in older patients. Rheumatoid arthritis affects the lining of the joints, and osteoarthritis affects the joint itself. When the lining is affected, there is more swelling. X-rays may also reveal joint deformity or even bone erosions.

Other Forms of Arthritis

While most patients know about the two most common forms of arthritis, osteoarthritis and rheumatoid arthritis, there are more than one hundred types in all.

The following list includes types of arthritis that are also well known:

- Psoriatic arthritis
- Reactive arthritis
- Ankylosing spondylitis
- Gout
- Fibromyalgia
- Degenerative disc disease
- Infectious arthritis
- Inflammatory arthritis
- Systemic lupus
- Metabolic arthritis

Other forms of arthritis that are autoimmune conditions are most often diagnosed in the younger population, but young patients tend not to take their symptoms as seriously as do elderly patients. However, if autoimmune conditions are not treated from the very beginning, they can lead to a lot of complications later.

Whenever a patient experiences these symptoms, their physician should definitely follow up with blood work every year. Most of these conditions are diagnosed through blood work, specifically autoimmune panels. Blood work can assist in diagnosing what form of arthritis is present, if it is a type other than osteoarthritis.

CHAPTER TWO

What Is the Standard of Care for Arthritis?

WHAT THE MEDICAL COMMUNITY PRE-SCRIBES FOR ARTHRITIS

Do you know how much money people in the United States spend annually on healthcare?

According to statistics made available by Pubmed.org, "National health expenditures will hit $3.35 trillion this year, which works out to $10,345 for every man, woman, and child. The annual increase of 4.8 percent for 2016 is lower than the forecast for the rest of the decade."[4]

The cost of healthcare is rising annually, with higher deductibles and larger premiums; however, do the treatments covered by our insurance actually work for us?

---

[4]Alonso-Zaldivar, Associated Press July 13, 2016

We will discuss how the medical community treats arthritis to give you a better understanding of how the most common treatments, such as medications or cortisone shots, do not address the problem of arthritis.

Consider these questions:

- When taking a pain medication, have you ever wondered how long you will continue to use it?

- Have you ever wondered why the pain starts up again as soon as you stop taking the pain medication?

- When you take a pain medication, are you are addressing only the symptoms, not the cause, of arthritis?

- If you don't address the cause of your pain, how are you going to be pain-free?

Even a cortisone shot does not address the cause of the problem: it addresses only the symptoms, and this temporary treatment is why arthritis persists.

The Medical Route for Treating Arthritis

When it comes to treating arthritis, the first option is to visit your family doctor or primary care physician.

What happens in that visit is that the doctor will most likely refer you to get an X-ray so that they can diagnose arthritis or see to what stage it has progressed. When that X-ray shows arthritic changes, then most of the time your doctor will prescribe a pain medication for relief of symptoms.

The problem with pain medications is they only mask the symptoms; they do not address the cause of the problem. This explains why, when a patient is placed on a pain medication, they will probably be taking that medication for the rest of their lives. This is a problem with arthritis because arthritis is also known as degenerative joint disease, and degenerative means the condition will worsen over time. As you are taking the pain medication and the process degenerates, the dosage will only increase as your arthritis progresses.

The other issue is that most medications have side effects. If you start developing side effects or new symptoms due to the use of pain medication, and you go back to your doctor with new symptoms, you will probably be placed on a new medication to treat the new symptoms.

A common over-the-counter drug that is used to treat pain is Tylenol, and its main ingredient is acetaminophen. Unfortunately, there have been many studies that prove that acetaminophen causes liver damage. Side effects and combinations with other prescriptions must be considered when you are given new medications.

What Pain Management Does for Arthritis

When you are referred to a pain management specialist, most of the time they will prescribe either an epidural injection or a cortisone shot. The problem with cortisone is that it is classified as a steroid; therefore, it has side effects. The most serious side effect of cortisone is that it causes bone softening or bone weakening. This is an issue because the most common type of arthritis is osteoarthritis, which is arthritis in the bones.

The other side effect is that cortisone raises sugar levels. Medicare covers only three cortisone injections per year because the side effects are serious and can lead to further complications. Cortisone will not address the cause of the problem; it will only mask the symptoms temporarily.

What Orthopedic Surgery Does for Arthritis

Often, when arthritis progresses to the point where it is affecting your daily activities or your quality of life, an orthopedic doctor will recommend surgery. The problem with this surgery is that it is not very successful. Some studies say that there is only about a 20 percent success rate when it comes to a lower back surgery. Also, when you get a knee replacement or have a knee surgery, knee replacements last for only ten years because the metal used to replace bone eventually wears out. Even after you get a surgery or some replacement, some patients still feel discomfort or pain because the surgery has not addressed the inflammatory portion that is generating pain.

The way most pain medications work is they block the pain pathway, from the area that is affected to the place in the brain that registers pain. What these medications do is to slow down the brain process. This can cause side effects such as:

- Cognitive impairment
- Increased memory loss

- Increased problems with balance
- Other issues

You need to keep in mind that while you are suffering from all these side effects, the medication is not really addressing the cause of the problem; it is simply working to mask the symptoms.

HOW THE STANDARD OF CARE TREATS ONLY THE SYMPTOMS OF ARTHRITIS

The United States makes up 5 percent of the world's population. However, at the present time, U.S. doctors prescribe 80 percent of the pain medications that are made around the world.

Almost all the patients who are on pain medications become addicted to them, and they are dependent on the medications for the rest of their lives. These patients don't understand the side effects of these medications and how they aren't really helping them, and in fact, because of side effects, the medications are actually causing patients greater harm.

The Physiology of Arthritis

Recall that the word *arthritis,* ends with *-itis,* which means *inflammation.* Therefore, arthritis is inflammation in the joints. When the standard of care prescribes a pain medication, it is not addressing the inflammation that is taking place. The inflammation that takes place is what limits the range of motion and causes pain, swelling, and decrease of mobility.

Even though you are on a pain medication and might be feeling a bit better, that joint, where you are still experiencing pain, is still inflamed. Therefore, that inflammation is not being addressed. The reason that this joint continues to deteriorate, even though you are taking a medication and you might be feeling better, is that as long as there is inflammation, the deterioration and progression of the condition will only continue.

Medications and Injections

Most of the patients we see in my practice have had cortisone injections or epidurals. Some say that the shots worked for them for a few months. Some say that the shots didn't work them for at all. The main thing to remember is that because of the way that these injections work, your arthritis will not be treated; instead, the pain from arthritis will be managed. Even if the injection worked for you in the short term, once you get an epidural or a cortisone shot, you are expected to go back and get another one.

Keep in mind that many patients suffer side effects from pain medications. Whenever you are placed on a drug, read about the side effects and learn how the drug can affect you. Most patients who are placed on these drugs will have side effects that could worsen the condition that is causing pain in the first place.

Ineffectiveness of Surgeries

Based on my experiences with treating osteoarthritis, surgery is not always the best option. Surgery can be effective in traumatic cases; however, when there is a systemic condition, performing surgery on L4–L5 in the lumbar spine, for example, will not stop arthritis from affecting the rest of the lumbar spine.

Some of my patients who are seeking treatment for their knees have already had their knees replaced, which means that they did not find the relief they were looking for and it did not take care of the problem for them.

There can be many complications from knee replacement surgeries:

- Staph infections
- Scar tissue buildup
- Knees not healing properly

Keep in mind that because arthritis is an inflammatory condition, surgery is not necessarily the answer.

Patients who have low back surgeries often need to go back for a second, third, or fourth operation because the degeneration of other discs in the spine was not addressed. Surgery, when it is successful, still works only in the specific place that the patient is complaining about or where they are experiencing pain at that time.

HOW MY TREATMENT ADDRESSES THE CAUSE OF THE PROBLEM

More than 80 percent of our patients usually find long-lasting relief in our treatment protocol. My recommendations are not merely short-term solutions—they are enduring changes.

I hope that everyone who is suffering from arthritis or knows someone who is suffering from arthritis comes to understand that there is another avenue for relief aside from the options that they have tried and that did not work for them. They don't have to stick to the standard of care that is failing to alleviate their condition. There is something else they can explore that can treat the causes of the problem and not simply work around the symptoms.

To be able to successfully treat the condition, it is important to restore circulation in the arthritic area to fight off inflammation. If there is an area of inflammation, that area is lacking oxygenated blood. Once oxygenated blood is restored in the inflammatory area, it accelerates tissue repair and cellular growth to repair the area.

The Treatment Protocol

Our arthritis treatments can vary based on the patient's state and what part of the body we are addressing. For example, most patients suffer from neck and low back arthritis. When cartilage starts to break down in the vertebrae or the bones, the bones start coming closer together, and that causes a lot of irritation and stiffness that tends to progress with the condition.

One thing we do in our treatment protocol is nonsurgical spinal decompression, which is also known as *traction*. The treatment gently pulls the spine and separates the vertebrae so that pressure is taken off the discs and the nerves. During spinal decompression, you are slowing down or stopping the progression of the condition and you are also treating the cause of the problem. Most of the pain is being generated from the compression of the discs and the nerves.

Another treatment I use is electrical stimulation which is a therapeutic modality. Many chiropractors, and even some medical doctors and physical therapists, use this modality to help treat pain in muscles or joint tissue. In this therapy, electrical stimulation is applied to prevent muscle atrophy. Two to four electrodes are applied to the skin, and the electrical stimulus helps the muscle contract.

This method also increases muscle strength and regeneration. It promotes proper muscle activity and strength.

Electrical stimulation helps in many conditions, such as:

- Tendinitis
- Tendinosis
- Muscle spasm
- Edema

It provides a great deal of help with arthritis because the muscle movement caused by electrical stimulation promotes an increase of blood circulation. Arthritis patients often experience decreased motor function, muscle atrophy, and difficulty walking. Throughout my years of practice, patients have experienced tremendous improvement in pain reduction, increased mobility, and increased strength through electrical stimulation.

How Laser Therapy Addresses Inflammation

The second step in our regimen is laser therapy. This therapy treats the cause of the problem by helping to increase the blood circulation in the area affected by arthritis. By increasing circulation, you push out inflammation.

Laser therapy simulates your body to build new blood vessels. There is a biological process called *angiogenesis*. *Angio* means *blood vessels*, and *genesis* means *growth*. By stimulating angiogenesis, or building new blood vessels in an area, you increase circulation. The reason this alleviates arthritis is because inflammation results from a lack of circulation.

When the laser treatment stimulates your body to build new blood vessels and increase circulation, you start pushing out the inflammation. You are then able to slow down or stop the progression of the condition, improve the symptoms overall, improve motion in the joint, and improve the patient's quality of life.

Results Are Long-Lasting, Because They Address the Cause of Arthritis

I have helped many patients who have tried physical therapy or exercise and have found temporary relief. When you are exercising or doing some sort of physical therapy, you are increasing circulation, but only temporarily.

However, with laser therapy, you are stimulating the body to build new blood vessels. These blood vessels are going to stay. We educate our patients on the specific diet program and certain exercises to help them maintain the integrity of those blood vessels. As long as the blood vessels remain, circulation will continue to bring oxygen and nutrients to that joint or area of the body.

These results are long lasting because you are actually making your body generate new blood vessels, in comparison to physical therapy or exercise, where you are only working with the blood vessels you have, which are not enough.

CHAPTER THREE

My Nonsurgical, Drug-Free Approach to Treating Arthritis

WHAT IS THE SECRET?

Many different treatments are offered for arthritis aside from the standard of care. It's important to explore and understand what is available that will treat the cause of the problem and not merely mask the symptoms. Understanding why this method is highly successful will help you to see how it could be helpful for someone who is suffering from or dealing with arthritis.

Decompression Therapy

Decompression therapy, also known as *nonsurgical spinal decompression* or *traction therapy*, is stretching of the spine by using a motorized traction table. This nonsurgical, drug-free procedure is highly successful at relieving spinal pain because it decreases the pressure that has been compressing the nerve. Once you relieve the pressure on the nerves that are shielded within the spinal discs, spinal pain subsides. Medications will mask the pain and yet not treat the cause of the pain, but nonsurgical spinal decompression directly treats the cause of the pain.

It is common for patients with arthritis to experience pain that radiates down the arms, which is caused by pressure to vertebrae in the neck, or pain that travels down their legs, which is caused by pressure in the lower back.

The pain can take many forms, such as:

- Numbness, tingling, or burning sensations
- Sharp, shooting pain or stabbing pain
- Coordination problems
- Balance problems

Once decompression therapy is applied to the neck or lower back, in most cases the pain that is traveling down the extremities begins to subside.

Decompression therapy is also helpful for degenerative joint disease and osteoarthritis, and for conditions such as:

- Herniated discs

- Bulging discs
- Sciatica

The goal of spinal decompression is to relieve pain and to restore the body to its optimal healing environment.

Laser Therapy

Laser therapy has many beneficial effects that help to relieve pain and, furthermore, also resolve inflammation. Laser therapy works by activating light photons that emit energy, and that energy is distributed over the area of the body that is being treated.

The laser activates photoreceptors in:

- Body tissues
- Muscles
- Tendons
- Ligaments
- Other body structures

There are many biological effects of laser therapy. The most important clinical effect of laser is angiogenesis, the development of new blood vessels. As mentioned earlier, by building new blood vessels, the body is capable of increasing blood circulation to the painful tissue. When you bring circulation in, inflammation is relieved, and the tissues start to heal themselves naturally. Increased blood flow helps to accelerate cellular reproduction growth, and also enables the cells to absorb more nutrients and eliminate waste products.

For example, a patient named Rebecca came to i-Spine Health Center with severe pain and swelling in her knees. She was diagnosed with osteoarthritis in both knees. The inflammation was severe, she had constant swelling, couldn't walk very far or stand for too long, kneel, go up and down stairs, or undertake ordinary, everyday chores.

Within only six sessions of laser therapy, Rebecca experienced a decrease in the swelling in both of her knees, which instantly decreased her pain and gave her greater range of motion.

I share this story with you because laser therapy treats the cause of the problem, which offers fast results, and can offer the swift success that Rebecca and many of our patients have experienced.

Biological Effects of Decompression and Laser Therapy

With traction treatment, different types of distraction forces are applied:

- Static
- Intermittent
- Cyclic

These distraction forces help to relieve pressure on structures such as nerves and discs that can be causing pain. When you distract the bones, they separate, so you are taking pressure off the disc and the nerve. In doing so, the nerve and the disc are allowed to slowly start to heal properly. This results in decreasing pain and decreasing symptoms that are generated from nerve compression, such as:

- Numbness
- Tingling
- Burning
- Sharp, shooting pains
- Balance problems

- Weakness
- Coordination problems

The biological effects that we observe from laser therapy are:

- Anti-inflammation
- Reduced pain
- Accelerated tissue repair and cell growth
- Improved vascular activity
- Increased metabolic activity
- Reduced fibrous tissue formation
- Improved nerve function
- Immune regulation

A study by Brian A. Pryor, PhD, offers the following conclusion:

> Tissue that is damaged and poorly oxygenated as a result of swelling, trauma, or inflammation has been shown to respond significantly to laser therapy irradiation. At the cellular level, deep penetrating photons activate a biochemical cascade of events leading to increased DNA/RNA, protein and collagen synthesis, increased cAMP levels, and cellular proliferation. The result of

these reactions is rapid cellular regeneration, normalization and healing. Laser light energy is highly absorbed by skin and subcutaneous tissue; therefore, penetration is key to therapeutic result. Longer wavelengths and higher power output result in deeper penetration and higher dosage to the tissue. Larger laser therapeutic dosage levels produce improved clinical outcomes as illustrated in the case and interventional studies cited above. LLLT (Classes I–III) does not provide optimal clinical outcomes in most disease conditions because they cannot deliver the necessary dosage to deep structures without using excessively long treatment times. Class IV lasers have been shown to provide both the wavelengths and output power levels necessary to trigger therapeutic cellular metabolic changes.[5]

The following list shows the different conditions that can benefit from laser treatment.

---

[5]Brian A. Pryor, "Class IV Laser Therapy: Interventional and Case Reports Confirm Positive Therapeutic Outcomes in Multiple Clinical Indications." Litecure.com. 2009.

Indications for Laser Therapy

Inflammatory Condition	Connective Tissue Injury/ Disorder	Joint Injury/ Disorder
Bursitis	Edema	Edema
Carpal Tunnel Syndrome	Effusion	Effusion of Joint
Edema	Inflammation	Inflammation
Effusion	Muscle Spasms	Ligament Injury
Epicondylitis	Myofasciitis	Osteoarthritis
Inflammation	Primary Diagnosis is Pain	Primary Diagnosis Pain in Joint
Muscle Spasms	Radicular Pain	Restricted Range of Motion/Stiffness
Myofasciitis	Restricted Range of Motion/Stiffness	Tempo-romandibular (TM) Disorders
Paresthesia	Sprains	
Plantar Fasciitis	Strains	
Primary Diagnosis Pain	Tendon Ruptures	
Radicular Pain	Tendonitis	
Restricted Range of Motion/Stiffness		

Rheumatoid Ar- thritis		

Pain Management	Muscle Injury/ Disorder	Neurological Injury/Disorder
Bursitis	Edema	Crush Injuries
Cervical/Neck Pain	Inflammation	Decreased Range of Motion/Stiffness
Edema	Muscle Bruises, Contusions	Edema
Effusion	Muscle Contractures	Effusion
Fasciitis	Muscle Ruptures	Inflammation
Fibro-myalgia	Muscle Spasms	Muscle Spasms
Inflammation	Myofasciitis	Myofasciitis
Low Back Pain	Myositis	Neuritis
Muscle Spasms	Primary Diagnosis is Pain in Joint	Paresthesia
Myofascial Pain	Restricted Range of Motion/Stiffness	Prolapsed Disk
Myofasciitis		Radicular Pain
Primary Diagnosis is Pain		Ruptured Disk

Restricted Range of Motion/Stiffness		Sciatica
Sciatica		Skin Injuries
		Edema
		Inflammation
		Post-operation: Incision, swelling, scar
		Pain in Joint
		Restricted Range of Motion/Stiffness
		Skin Grafts
		Skin Ulcers

THE FOUR PILLARS OF HEALTH

Patients often ask me if it is necessary to do the laser treatment again to maintain positive results. The answer is no. Understanding the four pillars of health allows you to participate in your own care and do your part to maintain the outcomes that you received from the treatment program every day for the rest of your life.

The four pillars of health are important to understand because when you support them, you promote better overall health, which includes reducing inflammation. Arthritis, as mentioned before, is an inflammatory condition. If the level of inflammation is lowered, then you are able to control arthritis as well as most diseases.

Laser therapy allows your body to promote angiogensis, and the new blood vessels created during this procedure are going to stay. This is how you maintain the results from the program, and it is not necessary to do the program again. However, you are responsible to maintain the integrity of the blood vessels through proper lifestyle, which includes diet and exercise. A diet that includes high levels of carbohydrates, sugars, and grain, can cause the blood vessels to become diseased and shriveled up, holding back proper circulation to joints. A good diet will allow the blood vessels to remain healthy, maintaining the positive results that you get out of the program.

For more guidance about how to support the best health, let's look at the four pillars of health in detail.

What Are the Four Pillars of Health?

Many people try to follow their doctor's advice about diet and exercise. However, many also feel they are not getting the results they are expecting. Most of the time, this occurs because they are not identifying the four pillars of health and treating each one separately. If you don't address all four pillars, you will most likely fail to see the results you are looking for.

As a wise man once said, "If you fail to prepare, you are preparing to fail." If you address two of the four pillars, which is what most people do, then you will receive only a small portion of the changes you are hoping to experience.

Let's take a closer look at the four pillars:

- Detoxification
- Nutrition
- Fitness
- Nervous system health

Unfortunately, in most doctor's offices, detox, fitness, and nutrition are rarely discussed.

Detoxification

By detoxing, you will allow your body to eliminate any waste products that are promoting more inflammation in the system.

Why Detox?

Detox means to clean out your body and blood. There are many benefits to detoxing and following a healthy diet. A detox combats diseases and decreases dependency on medications, such as those for blood pressure, diabetes, and high cholesterol. A healthy diet can also improve longevity, mood, energy, and mental health.

You are not expected to change your mindset and behavior overnight. You need to be patient and take it one day at a time. There are many forms of detoxing, some can start from fasting and drinking water only, or you can take supplements that are rich with natural herbs, or dieting.

The best form of detox is to clean up your diet.

Why is it important to detox?

An unhealthy lifestyle or diet leads to inflammation, where toxins start to affect normal body functions.

Have you ever asked yourself why you aren't losing weight if you're going to the gym, and you're trying and trying?

Most of the time that's because the body is unable to burn fat due to the high level of toxins in body, which causes your body to gain weight. Next, you start developing new diseases due to the weight gain such as diabetes, high blood pressure, and heart disease. When you detox, the goal is to get rid the toxins in your body that are stored in fat cells. Once you get rid of the toxins in your fat cells, metabolism increases.

When Should I Detox?

Detox is great if you're experiencing digestive issues such as IBS (Irritable Bowel Syndrome); an inflammatory condition, such as arthritis; or autoimmune conditions, such as thyroid, lupus, rheumatoid arthritis, psoriasis, and any other condition. Patients experiencing depression, mood swings, or even generalized fatigue usually have gastrointestinal inflammation, which is inflammation in the gut.

Detoxing usually helps increase brain function and decreases mood swings and depression. Even if you have no symptoms at all, to obtain optimal health it is best to detox twice a year. Detox not only cleans out the liver and promotes weight loss. but it helps reduce inflammation, boosts energy, and promotes proper skin health.

How Can I Detox Through Diet?

All you need to do is cut out sugar and grains.

Foods that you can eat include:

- Meats
- Fruits
- Fish
- Nuts
- Leafy greens
- Regional veggies
- Seeds

Focus on foods that energize, nourish, and burn fat:

- Red apples
- Avocado
- Blueberries

- Flax seed (Ask your doctor if you're on a blood thinner)
- Pomegranate
- Eggs
- Salmon
- Herbal teas

The first step is to cut out grains. Good news, there are alternatives to common grains. Health food stores, such as Whole Foods and Sprouts, carry almond bread, coconut bread, and sometimes you can find flaxseed bread. Rice can be substituted with quinoa, and pasta can be substituted with zucchini pasta and spaghetti squash.

An important part in detoxing is hydration. It is most effective to drink water equal to half of your body weight in ounces every day. That might seem like a lot of water in the beginning, but remember your blood is approximately 80 percent water.

Why eliminate sugar?

Sugar:

- Is found in almost all processed foods
- Increases chance of cardiovascular disease

- Can impair cognitive functions, including memory
- Lowers your immune system
- Increases depression and anxiety
- Is correlated with higher levels of cancers

Be sure to also stay away from artificial sweeteners.

They can lead to or aid in:

- Weight gain
- Depression
- Fatigue
- Arthritis
- Insomnia
- Rapid heart beat
- Memory loss
- Fibromyalgia
- Diabetes
- Birth defects

Substitute stevia for sugar and use organic honey in moderation.

The *No-No* List:

1. High fructose corn syrup—RUN, DON'T WALK!

2. Microwaves — They destroy molecules in food, making it unidentifiable to the body.

3. Aspartame, sucralose and saccharin — These kill brain cells (found in artificial sweeteners, diet sodas, candy, medications).

4. Protein bars — Use in emergencies only.

It is also important to check your vitamin D3 level. Vitamin D helps in reducing inflammation in the body; however, we need 8 hours of sunlight per day to make enough vitamin D3. As an industrialized nation, we do not get enough sunlight. Therefore, more and more patients are being diagnosed as vitamin D deficient.

Be sure to ask your doctor to check on your vitamin D3 level. If you are deficient in this crucial vitamin, it is easy to purchase a supplement at most drug stores. See your doctor for a recommended dosage.

Vitamin D3 deficiency can lead to:

- Osteoporosis
- Muscle aches and weakness
- Osteoarthritis
- High blood pressure
- Diabetes

It is also important to stay away from soy products. Soy consumption can lead to hormone irregularity. Also, soy products are usually a GMO (genetically modified organism), and are found in almost ALL boxed foods.

Soy can lead to:

- Breast cancer
- Food allergies
- Pregnancy complications
- Nervous system issues

Nutrition

Nutrition has a direct impact on your body. If you are eating the wrong foods, you can make your condition worse.

There are many diets that can be followed, but which one is the best diet to reduce inflammation and maintain a low inflammatory level?

An anti-inflammatory diet requires you to eliminate both grains and sugars from your meals. Sugars promote inflammation in the blood vessel wall by deteriorating the innermost layer of the blood vessel wall. This allows the buildup of scar tissue. Once the blood vessel is narrowed, it's going to decrease circulation of oxygen and nutrients to the tissue that is supposed to be fed. The body will respond with inflammation.

The problem with grains, such as bread, rice, and pasta, is that they spike your blood sugar level, and this promotes the inflammatory cycle. An alternative to avoiding grains entirely is to have bread made with almond flour and flaxseed flour, both of which can be found at julianbakery.com and other resources, such as Sprouts, Whole Foods, and Winco.

Fitness

A common misconception is that as long as you are exercising, you are doing fine. However, there are certain exercises that can aggravate arthritis or even make it more painful. When there is inflammation in the joint, the tissues that support the joint, such as muscles, become inflamed as well.

The muscles that support the joint become inflamed, and when we try to exercise with arthritis the activity can generate pain because we're working out inflamed muscles. I often hear from my patients that weight bearing exercises are painful. It is best to perform non-weight bearing exercises such as swimming or cycling.

This choice encourages an increase in blood circulating to the joints; however, there is no weight bearing down on the joint.

Fitness plays an important role because it is important for the spine and joints. By exercising and being in motion, blood circulation increases to benefit the joints, and this can help prevent further symptoms of arthritis or degeneration caused by the disease.

WHY IS THIS PROGRAM DIFFERENT?

My goal for all my patients is to not only to resolve your immediate problems, but also to see you graduate into a healthy lifestyle where you enjoy overall, everyday health. When you come to i-Spine for treatment, I incorporate fitness, nutrition, nervous system health, and detox into the program because this regimen will help you recover your health and improve your quality of life.

The patients who experience the greatest benefits from my treatment address their nutrition issues early, so that they are transitioning to that lifestyle while they are under our care. My staff and I make sure we are helping you to transition slowly and carefully, and that you are doing it the right way. I educate you on what to eat, what not to eat, what substitutes you can try, and how to eliminate certain foods. We also educate you on maintaining your results long after the treatment ends, by adhering to the four pillars of health.

CHAPTER FOUR

How Nutrition
Can Change Your Arthritis

WHAT IS AN ANTI-INFLAMMATORY DIET?

Diets are grouped into different categories, and an anti-inflammatory diet is a specific course of action with healthy ingredients. When it comes to dealing with an inflammatory condition, it's important to compare the standard American diet to other food habits around the globe. The more you understand what constitutes a good diet, the better you can take control of your condition.

The Standard American Diet

There are so many books and talks on dieting and nutrition that it is easy to be confused about which method will reduce inflammation. Furthermore, the standard American diet simply does not consist of healthy foods. This is a strong statement to make, but consider the main ingredients in typical American fare: dairy products, meat products, processed foods with high sugar content, and foods that are high in saturated fats.

Americans also fail to consume a good amount of vegetables and fruits, which are important in every diet.

Diabetes, obesity, heart disease, high cholesterol, high blood pressure, cancer, and Alzheimer's disease are all chronic conditions that are on the rise. Sadly, even the rate of childhood obesity is increasing every single year in the United States. We are becoming a sicker nation, at a faster pace, now more than ever before.

The United States is inundated with fast-food chains that offer poor-quality foods for very low prices. Healthful foods in this country are more expensive, making it difficult for individuals to afford organic produce, for example. In contrast, high-fat burgers in processed white buns are offered for low prices, and other processed foods are even cheaper. The cost of feeding a family is one reason Americans are failing to maintain good diets.

Defining the Anti-Inflammatory Diet

An anti-inflammatory diet is rich in fruits and vegetables. An anti-inflammatory diet begins with the elimination of grains and sugar and other foods that promote inflammation.

The list of foods to avoid includes:

- Empty carbohydrates
- Saturated fats
- Sugars
- Artificial sweeteners
- Grains
- Processed foods

Foods that you can eat include:

- Meats
- Fruits
- Fish
- Nuts
- Leafy greens
- Regional veggies
- Seeds

Most patients struggle with the prevalence and desire for grains: breads, rice, and pasta. Grains must be eliminated from the diet because of their negative impact when they are converted into high blood sugar in the body. Even though you feel that you are not eating a food that is high in sugar, grains are nevertheless a source of high blood sugar.

An anti-inflammatory diet is not followed mainly for losing weight; it is, instead, a way to gain more control over your body so that you can eliminate toxins from your system, which will eliminate inflammation and restore your body to a normal state of homeostasis.

How the Anti-Inflammatory Diet Affects Arthritis

Many patients who suffer from arthritis will notice that some days are better than others. This is mainly due to inflammation, which changes with diet and other factors. Patients who are highly sensitive will even notice that when they eat a particular food, their arthritis symptoms can worsen.

Another important reason why patients with arthritis should follow an anti-inflammatory diet is because by removing the cause of inflammation and reducing the inflammatory process in the body, your body can begin to heal itself naturally. Many patients with early stages of arthritis can possibly decrease their pain and slow down or stop the progression or degenerative process of arthritis through diet and proper supplement intake, especially the supplements that are needed for the specific place in their body that is affected.

THE EFFECTS OF THE ANTI-INFLAMMATORY DIET

My clinic is based on treating arthritis, and we have seen tremendous results in patients who have incorporated these anti-inflammatory diets into their lifestyles. They have experienced better results and have been able to maintain those results for longer periods of time, and we have also witnessed patients improving their health overall. Therefore, it is important to understand how effective this diet is and how it could have a huge impact on your health.

How Diet Directly Plays a Role on Inflammation

The word *chronic*, or *continuing a long time*, means that a process has been persisting for a while or recurs frequently. The longer that an inflammatory condition has been in the body, the longer there has been a lack of blood circulation. There is not enough blood flow within the system.

When you eat foods high in sugar and grains, they deteriorate the blood vessel wall, which can close the blood vessel completely and will limit circulation throughout your body. When you start eating properly, you stop that process from happening. You will allow it to increase circulation.

Oxygenated blood carries oxygen, nutrients, food, and water to your muscles, organs, and tissues to continually rejuvenate and heal your body. By maintaining a proper diet, you are directly fighting off the inflammation and are allowing the body to heal naturally.

Reduction in Inflammation Equals Reduction in Pain

When patients have arthritis at an early stage, they may wonder if they are experiencing more pain than others who are at a later stage in their arthritis. However, they can often experience less pain, and be more mobile that longer-term arthritis patients.

For example, a patient came to me with excruciating pain and a limited range of motion in her knees. She thought both knees were so degraded that bone was grating on bone. We took an x-ray and it showed that her knees were at a very early stage of degeneration. This patient was actually suffering from an autoimmune disorder, which caused a lot of inflammation.

When we were able to reduce the inflammation and take control of it through diet, supplements, and certain exercises, the pain in her knees reduced even though we did not treat her knees at all. Pain is a sign of inflammation. Pain is not necessarily a sign of a big or chronic condition.

Remember: the more you can control inflammation, the more you can control pain, as well.

How Inflammation Affects the Body Overall

I would like to share the story of my patient Inez. She came in with low back pain and pain in both knees, all due to arthritis. She had high blood pressure and high cholesterol, and she had been taking medications for these conditions for the past ten years.

We started a treatment program for her lower back and both of her knees. Inez took the diet very seriously, and she lost over forty pounds within a matter of eight weeks. The amazing result was that her blood work changed and showed such normal ranges that her primary doctor—the doctor who prescribed the high blood pressure and high cholesterol medications—told Inez that she no longer needed those medications.

All medications have side effects, and we never get better simply by being on medications, which treat symptoms and do not address the cause of the problem. However, the anti-inflammatory diet can have a positive overall effect on the body: it not only decreases inflammation, but can also normalize your blood work when conditions such as high cholesterol and high blood pressure are involved.

WHAT YOU CAN DO TO CHANGE YOUR DIET

Many people will begin a diet and then will stop after an average of four to six weeks. People tend to quit too easily when it comes to diets. One reason this occurs is because they start by depriving themselves, and change all their food habits within a day or two. This is not a positive way to begin a diet.

All it takes to change your diet is:

- Education regarding your condition
- Information on what you should eat, and what you should stay away from

- The positive mindset that you are ready to change your lifestyle
- The reasons for doing so

Taking control of your health and your life, and avoiding pain in the long run, are compelling reasons to change.

How to Create a Healthy Lifestyle

If we don't constantly work on our self-improvement, we only get worse over time. If you keep the same diet and it isn't healthy, your body will eventually deteriorate and experience pain. As you age, the food that you ate twenty years ago might begin to have a negative impact. Your metabolism changes, your cells change, and your body changes overall.

Starting a healthy lifestyle is not something you can do overnight. Most practitioners, doctors, and trainers don't expect their clients or patients to suddenly change the ways they have been eating and exercising overnight. Everyone understands it will take some time and proper education for you to change.

Learn What Is Good for You

The first step is education. Once you are educated regarding what is good for you and what to avoid, you can start implementing these changes slowly. When you start introducing more healthy foods into your diet, you will begin to feel better, and you may notice a difference in your body. One of the biggest changes noticed by a lot of my patients is that the swollen feeling in their arms, legs, and trunk begins to go away. This kind of change helps you become more motivated, and it helps you keep going on to the next step.

I always tell my patients that it is important to look at their blood work because it will tell us which supplements are best and which ones to stay away from. You also might be sensitive to certain kinds of foods. A good way to begin treatment is to get a comprehensive blood work panel to see where you stand. Based on this, you can see what you are sensitive to and what is harmful for you.

How to Eliminate Grains and Sugars

A basic and immediate change I advise my patients to take is to eliminate fast foods and to cut out soda. An average soda has thirteen to fourteen teaspoons of sugar. Eliminating fast foods is important because they are very high in processed sugar, and that processed sugar creates toxins in your body.

Processed sugar has the following effects:

- Causes you to gain weight
- May have unforeseen side effects
- Makes you more susceptible to *hyperglycemia*, or an excess of sugar in the blood, that can lead to diabetes

When you start to eliminate foods that have a negative impact on your system, you will begin to notice a difference, and the changes will become self-motivating because you will want to continue.

The biggest problem for most of my patients is eliminating sugars because they use sugar with their coffee or tea in the morning and in other drinks throughout the day. Our American diet offers artificial sweeteners such as Splenda, Sweet 'n Low, or Equal. Unfortunately these are neurotoxins, meaning they cause toxicity to brain cells. Their side effects are horrendous, from numbness to weight gain to skin rashes. Some of these artificial sweeteners can even cause Alzheimer's disease or tremors.

According to research presented in *Environmental Health Perspectives*:

> If mice are given aspartame in doses that elevate plasma phenylalanine levels more than those of tyrosine (which probably occurs after any aspartame does in humans), the frequency of seizures following the administration of an epileptogenic drug, pentylenetetrazole, is enhanced. This effect is simulated by equimolar phenylalanine and blocked by concurrent administration of valine, which blocks phenylaline's entry into the brain. Aspartame also potentiates the induction of seizures by inhaled fluorothyl or by electroconvulsive shock. Perhaps regulations concerning the sale of food additives should be modified to require the reporting of adverse reactions and the continuing conduct of mandated safety research.[6]

The easiest way to reduce the use of sugar without using artificial sweeteners is to switch to stevia. Stevia

---

[6]Maher, T.J. and R.J. Wurtmen. "Possible neurologic effects of aspartame, a widely-used food additive." *Environmental Health Issues* 75 (November 1987). Ncbi.nlm.nih.gov/pmc/articles/PMC1474447/.

is an organic sweetener that is widely available. It is derived from the stevia plant and is marketed under several different brand names. You can find it in a powder or a liquid form.

However, when it comes to grains, the main problem for our patients is bread. Bread is everywhere in the American diet, and is usually made from whole wheat or more heavily processed wheat (white) flour.

What are the kinds of breads that we can consume?

There are breads made from almond flour, coconut flour, and flaxseed flour. These breads can easily be found at grocery stores or even online. Or, you can make them at home yourself. There are recipes accessible on the web that can help you prepare any of these breads.

All it takes to follow a diet is the mindset and determination to do so. Most of my patients are able to eliminate grains and sugars within three to four weeks. They tell me that the changes were not a big problem and were entirely doable. It takes two weeks to establish a habit, so once you are able to eliminate grains and sugars, you are going to notice that you really don't need them as much as you thought you did.

The Anti-Inflammatory Diet Is Easy to Follow

The biggest misconception about diets and why many people believe they don't work is because a timeline is placed on them. In order to follow a diet, you have to forget the timeline and approach it as a lifestyle change. Lifestyle changes don't happen overnight, and you can't expect to change your life drastically and the way you've been eating overnight. It will take time, dedication, and willpower. And it does take some time for you to educate yourself about what is good for you and what is not.

There is a famous quote that I like to share with my patients: "If you really want to do something, you will find a way. If you don't, you will find an excuse."

This quote is very powerful because if you are really dedicated, you develop the right mindset, and if you really want to change your quality of life, you will be able to change.

It takes planning. An effective way to make changes is to come up with a plan or schedule every week of what you are going to have for breakfast, lunch, and dinner.

If you plan your menu week by week, and you have a schedule and are able to prepare these meals, then it is not too difficult to follow.

In the beginning, it is normal to have withdrawal symptoms as you remove foods from your diet. It is normal to feel like giving up, but that is the time to look for support, which is always available.

You can look toward these sources for support:

- Doctors
- Trainers and coaches
- Friends
- Members of an online or community group

Most of my patients struggle in the first few weeks of the diet, but with support they get through the transition. Then, they see the bigger picture and how much value there is in changing their lifestyle to something better.

The main goal is being healthy. Once you notice how healthy you feel when you cut out bad foods, you will have more motivation to follow through with this diet. You will tell all your friends that it is really not that difficult to follow this diet.

CHAPTER FIVE

Patient Testimonials

My quality of life has improved to the point where I can walk and sit without experiencing excruciating back pain. In addition, I am able to sleep well at night. Pain level in back has gone from a 4 or 5 to a 2 or 3. The latter varies from a low 2 in the mornings to sometimes a high 3 in the late afternoon. Overall, I experienced a huge improvement.

~ Armando

I came into i-Spine Health Center because I was experiencing great pain all the time in my lower back. The pain was constant throughout the day and even more so through the night. Prior to coming here, I had tried injections; they were a temporary fix. The doctors I was seeing wanted to operate, which I said no to. That is when I started researching ways to help stop the pain. That is when I found Dr. A. and his seminars. Since starting treatment here I feel as if I am a new person all because of Dr. A. and the treatments he provides. I am now free of back pain. I am more mobile, I sleep better, and am able to sit and stand without the normal sharp shooting pain I would experience. When asked if I would refer family and friends here my answer will always be yes, yes, and more yes!

~ Brenda 1

The reason I decided to become a patient at i-Spine Health Center was because I was having terrible pain in my knee and low back. What really caught my attention was during the dinner talk when the doctor mentioned wall walking throughout my house for support. Previously I had tried talking to my primary doctor and was prescribed medication and referred to useless physical therapy. I was not skeptical about trying a new treatment, I was just concerned I would get no relief, but that was not the case. The two benefits I saw immediately were more energy and flexibility, which I thought I had lost forever. The benefits and positive impact this treatment has had on my life is being able to move with less discomfort. I am baking again, and my projects are moving along much faster than usual. Overall I seem to be doing and feeling better.

~ Brenda 2

I attended the presentation at Cocos in Covina. When I heard the doctor talking about arthritis and how he could help, I knew there could be help for me. I came to the office seeking help for my back pain and nerve pain in my toe. Laser therapy and decompression therapy have helped me a lot. Prior to coming here, I tried pain medications, which were a temporary fix, not a cure. I would have to take five pills to feel any relief from the pain in my toe. Since starting treatment at i-Spine Health Center I am now able to do more housework and shopping with less pain and stiffness. I have little to no nerve pain in my toe now, which allows me to wear almost any shoes I'd like, and I am also able to go dancing again with no issues. I am more than happy and have already been referring friends and family to come for treatment. I have to thank the wonderful girls at the center for their kindness and care they have given me. God bless you, Dr. A. and your staff.

~ Catherine

Before coming to i-Spine Health Center I experienced neck pain that extended all the way down to my shoulder blades. The pain prevented me from turning my head or twisting my neck. For example, when I was driving I had a hard time looking to either side in both directions. Now when I drive I feel much safer. My neck pain has gone down and my range of motion is not restricted. The shooting pain in my shoulder blades has also gone down. My quality of life had changed 100 percent. I feel so much more energetic. Now that I don't have the pain I want to be more active and do different things that I wasn't able to do before. For anyone that is considering treatment here, I would tell them to give it a try and not to hesitate!

~ Carmen

Charles had lower back pain for years and since starting Dr. A's treatments it has disappeared.

He can do things now that he hasn't been able to do in years.

My bursitis has lessened in pain since starting treatments as well. And I am able to walk for longer periods of time without the pain. We feel so great that we are going on a cruise!

~ Charles and Ruth

The treatment itself felt good — decompression, electrical stimulation, and laser. The results were a gradual and steady decrease in pain in both hips and increased mobility. These contributed to more energy and activity and even more improvement in mood. I am so grateful to be relieved of four years of chronic pain and very limited activity. Dr. Al-Selhi, Kirstin and Alex are always friendly and attentive.

~ Cindy

Since starting treatment, not only has the pain in both of my knees decreased a lot, but the tingling sensation also went away completely. The tingling was so bad that it would keep me up at night and would be so uncomfortable. Walking does not bother me at all anymore either and going up and down the stairs has gotten much easier for me as well. It only took three treatments for me to notice a positive change in my pain levels. In addition to my knee, I was always getting headaches. Dr. A. started to do neck decompression treatments for me. After the first treatment, my headaches stopped and have not came back. I am very happy with my treatment.

~ Coleta

No more constant pain or the terrible aches and pain due to bad weather. I can go on my walks without worrying about walking down a hill (since that was most painful before treatment). I'm hustling all over the place, pain-free. I would recommend everyone to go through this treatment before considering surgery. I know it will be successful.

~ Connie

I suffered from chronic neck and back pain for over twenty years. I had many procedures to help relieve the pain, which include chiropractic care, adjustments, cortisone shots, trigger points, and *many prescribed pain medications. My sister saw one of the ads in the paper and called me right away to attend one of the seminars because she knew that I had tried many things before that hadn't worked. I was skeptical about seeing another doctor, but I learned a lot about my condition after attending the dinner seminar and was interested in seeing if I qualified for care at i-Spine Health Center. The benefits I received from Dr. A.'s office are that I have been able to reduce my pain pill intake, I can walk further distances without having to stop so often because of pain, and I can do more activities than I have in a long time. The pain in my neck and back has gone down quite a bit. I enjoyed the staff so much I felt that I had made friends, not simply seeing office personnel, when I came in for my treatments. I look forward to seeing everyone in the office and I appreciate how sweet and courteous everyone is. I have enjoyed coming in to i-Spine Health Center because they are such a friendly, fun group of people. I always feel comfortable being in their company. I would recommend this treatment because it is so different than the other treatments being offered because Dr. A. fixes the problem instead of masking it with pills, adjustments, and shots.*

~ Dee

I was diagnosed with osteoarthritis. I had pains and stiffness in my neck and back and I think the treatments have helped me in certain movements. I started feeling positive changes about halfway through my treatment. If you have the time and money to invest in your own personal health, such as I did, I would recommend it.

~ Edward

When I first came to i-Spine Health Center I was experiencing sciatic pain that radiated down the back of my legs all the way down to my feet. I really didn't have any other problems aside from that. Before my treatment I was unable to do some of my housework and any time I had to bend over I would experience electric shocks down my legs and thighs. The pain was so bad that it would make me cry. That's when I started to seek help. After starting treatment here I felt much better. I noticed a lot of improvements, not only to reduce my pain but also to improve my health. Being on the diet has tremendously helped because I've lost so much weight and am continuously losing. My quality of life has improved; housework is easier and I can finally enjoy time with my grandkids. It has been a gratifying experience. Dr. A. has been awesome. I would highly recommend this treatment. I would urge people to do treatment here. They will truly experience a positive change in their pain and life.

~ Inez

After ten treatments I have days when I have only two or three short periods of pain, but I have had several days of no pain at all. Before treatment I was experiencing pain almost continually most days. I never had days without shooting pain in my back and burning pain in my leg. I am looking forward to continuous improvement with my treatments here.

~ Janice

I came for treatment on my lower back, knees, shoulders, and neck. My shoulder pain is completely gone and my other symptoms have also improved. My shoulder pain was so bad that

I would cry, and it kept me from getting a good night's sleep. Now I am without pain and am able to function through life so much better.

~ Josephine

The reason I came to i-Spine Health Center was because I was looking for ways to alleviate discomfort, which in my particular case was in my knees. I saw the ad in the paper and I decided to attend one of the seminars to get more information. I had never been to a chiropractor before, but a doctor in internal medicine told me my condition was due to the aging process, so I was looking for ways to lower the pain I was having in my knees, ankles, and in the soles of my feet. After coming for treatment at i-Spine Health Center, the pain I mentioned decreased and I was able to sleep through the night without pain. It lessoned my anticipation of lasting pain, and increased my ability to walk longer distances with less pain. My overall experience has been great. Everyone is very thoughtful and generous with advice and offering me water. The reason I tell people to come to my chiropractor is because of the short time it took to see results with the laser treatment. My leg pain no longer exists, and my sleep and walking has improved.

~ Louise

The reason I came to i-Spine Health Center was because I have arthritis in my right knee. Prior to coming to i-Spine I tried pain medications and stem cell therapy, which worked temporarily for a few months. After having no luck with what I had tried previously, Dr. Al-Selhi started treating my knee. Within a few sessions of laser therapy and electrotherapy, my pain started to decrease, and I started walking and eating better. I am now being treated for peripheral neuropathy in my lower legs and feet, which has really improved. I refer my friends and family to i-Spine Health Center because I tell them that Dr. Al-Selhi and his team do a great job listening and treating their patients. Before coming to i-Spine Health Center, it was very hard to for me to walk and now I have been walking about four blocks at a time. Overall my experience here at i-Spine Health Center has been great!

~ Marjorie

Before treatment I had constant levels of pain of a 3 or 4 when I got up, and throughout the day the pain would go up and down depending on my daily activity. The changes I've had are that I now have little to no pain throughout most of my day. It only took about four or five days for me to notice a change in the pain. I am a happy camper now.

~ Marly

When I first started treatment at i-Spine Health Center, I had pain in my neck and my back. I was unable to turn my head while driving, I had slow mobility, and I was unable to do regular activities without extreme pain. From experience, physical therapy did not help with the pain I had in my back. When I first started I was extremely eager to get help, and by the second week the pain was down 50 percent and I was much more easily able to do things around the house. I went to an event and I was unaware I would have to walk a distance, and when I later returned home I realized that without this treatment, that walk would not have been possible. What I would say to someone considering treatment here is that if you are considered as a candidate for care, don't hesitate. The possibility that I could benefit from this was a chance I was willing to take, not just for myself but also for my family, because ending up in a wheelchair was not an option for me. Dr. A. and his staff made my treatment understandable and enjoyable.

~ Mary Lou

I noticed a big change, especially doing household work. I can do 80 to 90 percent of the work that needs to be done, while before I could only do 50 percent. Thanks, Dr. A., Kirstin, and Alex.

~ Nancy

I signed up for treatment here at i-Spine, and since starting treatment I am not as stiff or in as much pain. I am happy with the results. Spinal decompression and laser treatment have made positive changes in my life. I've had a positive experience and definitely recommend it to those suffering from stiffness.

~ Richard

I am thankful to have done this treatment. When I started I was taking a lot of pain medications, which still didn't take the pain away. Now I am virtually pain-free with an occasional all-day pain reliever. I no longer need a cane or knee brace. I can now easily ascend and descend the stairs normally with both feet and sometimes at a sprint. Thank you, Dr. A.

~ Rosa

I originally came into I-Spine Health Center for the discomfort I had been having in my back and legs, I had difficulty walking and my feet always felt puffy. After attending the seminar, I felt that the treatment could give me some relief. At first I was a little skeptical as I had previously had different treatments for my condition and it only helped a little, but never increased my comfort very much. Since starting my treatment at i-Spine, the pain in my lower back is now gone. I am able to sleep better and family outings and church, which were always a priority regardless of my condition, are now easier to do. My overall experience here has been excellent. Dr. A. and the staff are great and always keep us comfortable.

~ Shirley

The main reason I came into I-Spine Health Center was for the pain I was having in my left knee. It was very limiting, I couldn't stand or put weight on it, it would also go out from under me from time to time. Prior to coming in, I had tried hot packs and cold packs, neither of which helped. Since starting treatment here, the pain in my knee was gone after my very first treatment. I noticed that I could stand, walk, and move more easily and without pain. Had I not started treatment here, I knew I would be using a walker. I overall enjoyed every treatment and the staff here.

My advice for people considering this type of treatment: "Why be in pain? This may be different, but it works!"

~ Sarah

I came to i-Spine Health Center to get relief from my back pain. I have arthritis in the spine and I don't like taking pain meds. I was skeptical at first, but during the first few treatments I noticed the pain decreasing, especially in the morning when I wake up. Unless I do heavy housework or stand for many hours, I'm almost pain-free most days. My quality of life has improved, my pain has decreased considerably, and I've recommended this treatment to my friends and family. Overall my experience at i-Spine has been great. Dr. A., Kirstin, and Alex are so friendly and caring. A really great team!

~ Silvia

Once I found out that I had DDD, I decided to do some research and the iSpine Center was recommended. I came in for a free consultation and they said they could help me with the pain I was in. I started the treatments and they were absolutely right. My pain has greatly diminished and I can get my life back. Everyone at the center was always so nice, willing to answer any questions I may have had at any time, at any stage in my treatment course. Everyone here at the center was always so professional. I would recommend checking out this center for back pain, no matter what the pain is from.

Thank you so much for everything!

~Susan G.

Conclusion

Throughout this book, we have discussed the condition of arthritis and by now you have a clear idea of what the U.S. standard of care is and how nutrition plays a role in the level of inflammation in our bodies. Our best defense against arthritis is to promote awareness of the disease and the many approaches that can be taken to stop and even to reverse this condition.

We need to let our friends and family and support groups know all about the new methods to treat arthritis. The more we are aware of what choices are available and what else can be done, the more we can achieve.

I urge you to share this book with others:

- People who suffer from arthritis
- People who are curious about alternative medicines
- People who want to understand the current healthcare system in the United States
- People who want to learn about inflammation and the anti-inflammatory diet

By sharing this book, you will be able to help more and more people, and we will be able to move forward as a nation toward better healthcare. Our purpose is to begin a movement, because our healthcare system is treating only the symptoms, and failing to treat the causes, of arthritis and other conditions. Every single movement in history started with one person, and that one person could possibly be you.

By sharing our experiences, we can achieve better healthcare for ourselves and for this nation overall.

Next Steps

Visit our website today—iSpineHealthCenter.com—to see if you qualify for a free evaluation with Dr. Al-Selhi, or call our office at 626-335-4466 to find out about our dinner events.

About the Author

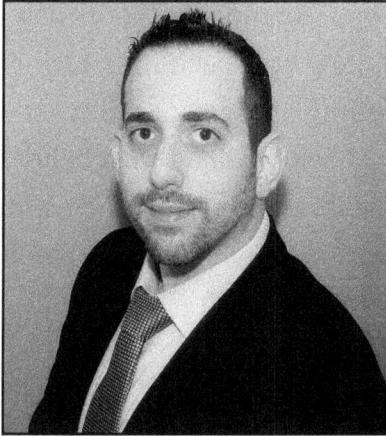

Fadi G. Al-Selhi, Doctor of Chiropractic (DC), is a licensed Chiropractic Physician in the state of California and Clinic Director of i-Spine Health Center. Dr. Al-Selhi specializes in treating arthritis, back pain, joint pain, personal injuries, and rehabilitation.

Dr. Al-Selhi obtained his Doctorate of Chiropractic Degree from Cleveland Chiropractic College, Los Angeles. Prior to obtaining his chiropractic degree, he graduated from California State Polytechnic University, Pomona, with a Bachelor's of Science Degree in Biology.

Dr. Al-Selhi believes there is never a time to stop learning, so he is currently continuing his education at Carrick Institute for Graduate Studies, completing a diploma in Functional Neurology. Functional neurology is a new approach for treating neurological disorders without the use of any medications or surgeries. Dr. Al-Selhi is also a member of the American Chiropractic Association, which helps him to stay up to date on what's new in the field so that he can deliver the best to his patients.

His goal is to provide state-of-the-art, nonsurgical, drug-free treatments to relieve pain.

In his free time, Dr. Al-Selhi enjoys hiking with his wife and four-year-old son and studying different plants. Dr. A also enjoys taking his son to the beach, so they can search together for marine organisms. On Sundays, he spends time with his family at church and volunteers as much as possible.